UNVEILING HEPATITIS B

NAVIGATING THE SILENT INTRUDER

RANDY SARA

Hepatitis B symptoms

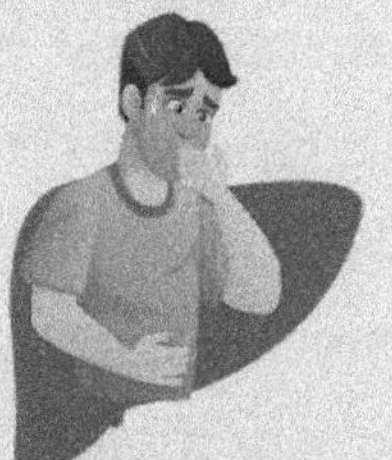

1. Nausea

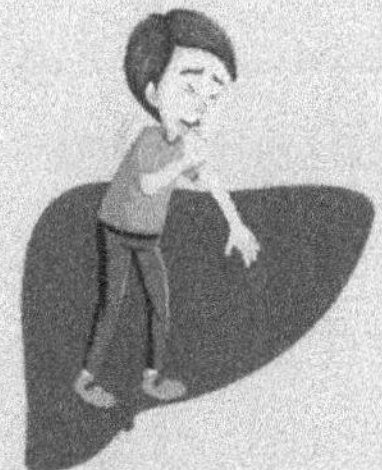

2. Vomiting

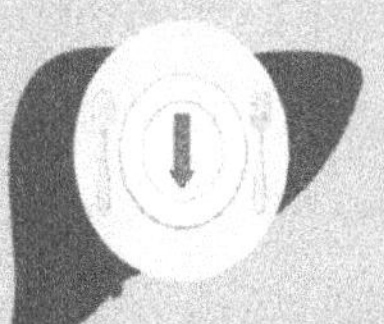

3. Loss of appetite

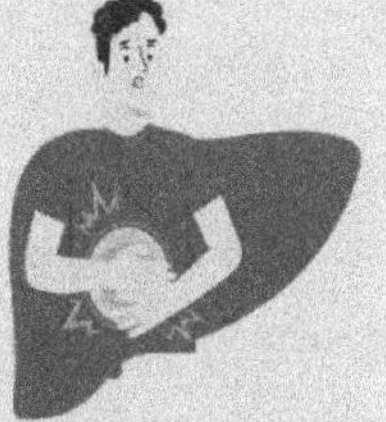

4. Pain in abdomen

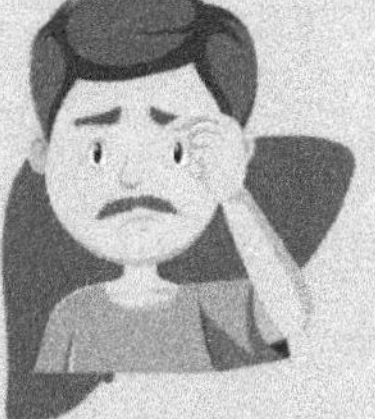

5. Jaundice

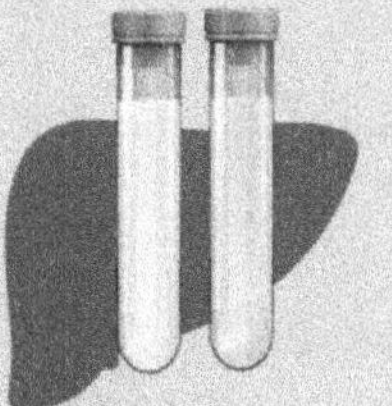

6. Dark urine

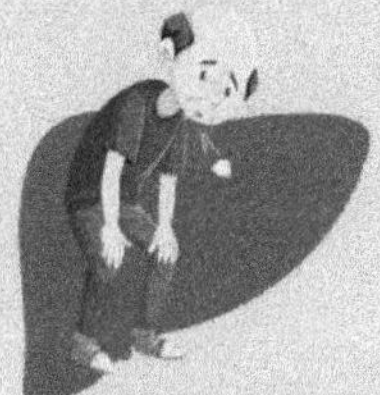

7. Tiredness

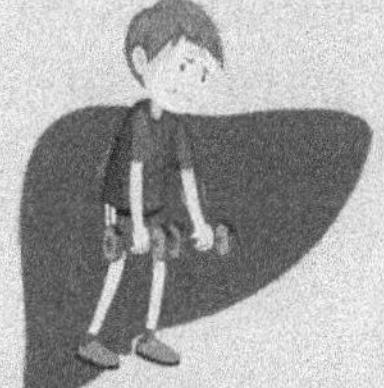

8. Weakness

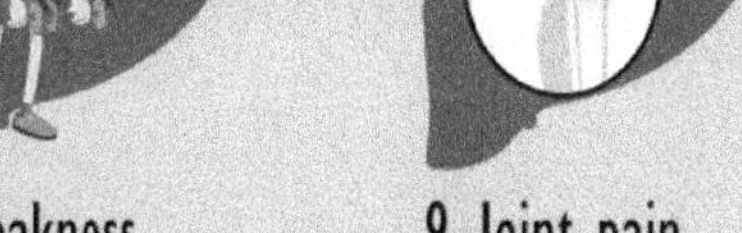

9. Joint pain

www.sprintmedical.in

INTRODUCTION

AN OVERVIEW OF THE B VIRUS

A viral infection that mostly affects the liver, hepatitis B can result in both acute and chronic liver disease and is brought on by the hepatitis B virus (HBV). Contact with infected blood, sperm, or other body fluids can spread the virus. With an estimated 257 million people worldwide living with chronic hepatitis B infection, it is a major global health issue.

History

Even though the hepatitis B virus was only discovered in the 1960s, hepatitis B has been recognized as a distinct disease for centuries. A significant step forward in the fight against hepatitis B was the creation of a vaccine in the 1980s. In many parts of the world, the prevalence of hepatitis B has significantly decreased as a result of the vaccine's effectiveness in preventing the disease.

Impact on the World

Globally, hepatitis B is a significant issue for public health. It is widespread, particularly in East Asia, the Pacific Islands, and sub-Saharan Africa. The disease's burden varies from country to country and population to population, with high prevalence rates in some areas.

Hepatitis B has a significant impact on both individuals and communities. Fatigue, nausea, and jaundice are all symptoms of acute hepatitis B infection. While most adults who get acute hepatitis B recover completely, a significant number of children who get it develop chronic hepatitis B, which can cause problems for a long time.

Inflammation of the liver (hepatitis), liver cirrhosis (scarring), liver failure, and an increased risk of liver cancer are all possible outcomes of chronic hepatitis B infection. Worldwide, hepatitis B is the leading cause of liver cancer. Hepatitis B complications, such as cirrhosis and liver cancer, are responsible for approximately 887,000 deaths annually, according to estimates.

The prevention of hepatitis B through vaccination, screening and diagnosis, and access to treatment have been the primary focuses of efforts to combat it. Numerous nations have implemented vaccination programs, resulting in significant decreases in the number of new infections. Reaching vulnerable populations, ensuring universal vaccination coverage, and facilitating affordable testing and treatment remain obstacles.

It is essential to control the spread of hepatitis B, improve outcomes for those who have it, reduce stigma and discrimination, and encourage early diagnosis and timely treatment. The goal of global initiatives like the World

Health Organization's Global Hepatitis Program is to make it easier for people all over the world to access services like testing, prevention, and treatment for hepatitis B.

Even though hepatitis B remains a significant global health issue, vaccination, education, and improved healthcare services have made progress in combating the disease. However, to achieve effective hepatitis B prevention, diagnosis, and treatment for all populations, ongoing efforts are required.

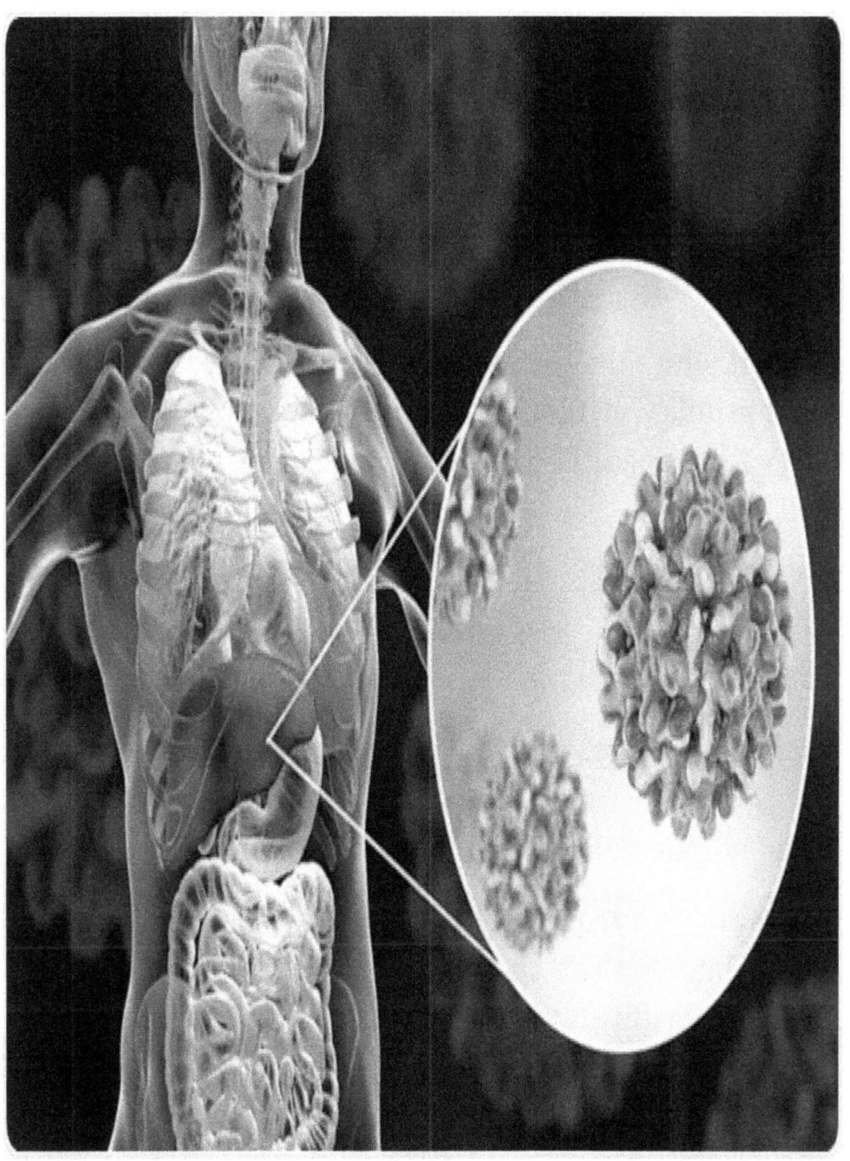

CHAPTER ONE
TRANSMISSION, VIRUS'S STRUCTURE, AND ITS EFFECTS ON THE LIVER

Transmission

Contact with infected blood, sperm, or other bodily fluids is the primary method by which the hepatitis B virus (HBV) is spread. The most prevalent transmission methods are:

<u>Sexual Activity</u>: Sexual contact without protection from an infected person can spread HBV. Sexual contact, whether oral or vaginal, can spread it.

<u>Sharing Syringes and Needles</u>: The virus can be spread through the sharing of contaminated needles or other drug paraphernalia, such as spoons or syringes.

<u>Transmission from Mother to Child</u>: During labor, an infected mother can transmit HBV to her unborn child. During breastfeeding, an infected mother can also spread the virus to her child.

<u>Blood that has been infected</u>: Transmission can occur through direct contact with infected blood, such as through needle stick injuries, blood transfusions (which are uncommon in nations with strict blood screening procedures), or the use of contaminated medical equipment.

Other Options: Although it is less common, close personal contact with an infected person, such as sharing razors or toothbrushes, can transmit HBV.

Virus Organization:

The Hepadnaviridae family includes the hepatitis B virus. It carries its genetic material in the form of DNA because it is a virus with partially double-stranded DNA. The envelope, or outer shell, of the virus, is made up of proteins called surface antigens (HBsAg). The nucleocapsid, which houses the viral DNA, enzymes, and core antigens (HBsAg), is located within the envelope.

The hepatitis B virus is extremely durable, and it can survive outside the body for up to seven days. It is an effective transmitter because of its durability, which helps it survive and remain infectious.

Symptoms for the Liver:

The liver is the primary organ that is infected with hepatitis B, and complications that are related to the liver can occur. The virus infects liver cells when it enters the body, causing inflammation and tissue damage to the liver.

People may experience fatigue, abdominal pain, loss of appetite, joint pain, nausea, vomiting, and jaundice (yellowing of the skin and eyes) in acute cases. Within six months, most adults infected with acute hepatitis B completely recover. However, acute infection can sometimes progress to chronic hepatitis B, which is when the virus remains in the body for more than six months. It may result in ongoing inflammation of the liver, which may eventually lead to cirrhosis and fibrosis (scarring) of the liver. A late-stage liver disease called cirrhosis is characterized by extensive scarring, liver structure disruption, and impaired liver function.

Chronic hepatitis B patients are also more likely to experience complications like liver failure and hepatocellular carcinoma (HCC), a kind of liver cancer. People who already have cirrhosis have a greater chance of developing liver cancer.

It is essential to keep in mind that not everyone who has chronic hepatitis B will develop severe liver disease. Various factors, including age at infection, immune response, and preexisting medical conditions, influence the progression and severity of the infection.

Living with chronic hepatitis B necessitates regular liver function testing and screening for liver cancer. Early diagnosis, appropriate medical management, and antiviral treatment can help slow the progression of liver disease and lower the risk of complications.

SYMPTOMS AND DIAGNOSIS
COMMON SYMPTOMS EXPERIENCED BY PEOPLE INFECTED WITH HEPATITIS B.

People who have hepatitis B can experience a variety of symptoms. It's important to remember that not everyone infected with the virus will show symptoms, especially in the beginning, when the infection is at its most severe. However, symptoms can include the following:

Fatigue: enduring feelings of exhaustion, fatigue, and lack of energy.

Pain in the Abdomen: Pain or discomfort in the liver's location in the upper right quadrant of the abdomen.

Appetite Suppression: a decreased appetite or a noticeable reduction in food intake.

Vomiting and vomiting: exhibiting symptoms of nausea or vomiting.

Jaundice: eyes and skin turning yellow. This occurs because the damaged liver is unable to effectively process the buildup of bilirubin, a yellow pigment produced during the breakdown of red blood cells.

<u>Urine Color:</u> Due to elevated bilirubin levels, urine may appear dark or tea-colored.

<u>Stools of Pale:</u> Due to a decrease in bilirubin production, stool may turn pale or clay-colored.

<u>Joint Pain:</u> numbness or pain in the joints, frequently accompanied by stiffness.

<u>Fever:</u> a slight to moderate rise in body temperature.

<u>Influenza-like Side effects:</u> A low-grade fever, headache, and other flu-like symptoms may occur in some individuals.

It is essential to keep in mind that the severity of these symptoms can vary and may not be present in all cases. In addition, symptoms alone are not sufficient to diagnose hepatitis B because they may also be indicative of other diseases. It is essential to seek medical attention and undergo testing for an accurate diagnosis if you suspect you have been exposed to hepatitis B or are experiencing any of these symptoms.

DIAGNOSTIC METHODS USED TO DETECT THE VIRUS

Blood tests that look for specific markers associated with the virus are typically used in diagnostic methods for hepatitis B virus (HBV) infection. These tests help determine the stage and activity of the infection, as well as whether a person has acute or chronic hepatitis B. Some common diagnostic techniques include:

Test for the Hepatitis B Surface Antigen (HBsAg): The hepatitis B virus's surface protein, HBsAg, is detected by this test. It is the most common way to check for hepatitis B. If HBsAg is found in the blood for more than six months, this means that you have chronic hepatitis B.

Core Antibody (anti-HBc) Test for Hepatitis B: This test does not differentiate between acute and chronic infection, so additional tests are typically required to determine the stage of the infection. The presence of anti-HBc antibodies indicates prior or ongoing infection with hepatitis B.

Anti-HBs Hepatitis B Surface Antibody Test: This test looks for antibodies that are made after getting the hepatitis B vaccine or after recovering from an earlier infection. Hepatitis B e Antigen (HBeAg) Test: If anti-HBs are found, this means that the person is immune to hepatitis B. HBeAg is a sign that the virus is actively reproducing and is highly infectious. Its presence indicates a greater likelihood of infection transmission to others. Patients with chronic hepatitis B frequently undergo HBeAg testing to evaluate disease activity.

<u>Test for Hepatitis B DNA (viral load):</u> The amount of HBV DNA in the blood is measured by this test. It helps determine the stage of infection as well as the patient's response to treatment and provides information about the level of viral replication. A more active infection typically indicates a higher viral load.

<u>LFTs (liver function tests):</u> The liver's function and damage are measured by these blood tests, which measure a variety of enzymes and substances. LFTs can be used to monitor the progression and severity of liver disease.

To determine the extent of liver damage, fibrosis, or the presence of liver cancer, additional tests like a liver biopsy or imaging procedures like an ultrasound, CT scan, or MRI may be recommended in some instances.

Counseling medical care proficiency for legitimate testing and understanding of the results is significant. To arrive at an accurate diagnosis and devise an appropriate treatment strategy, they will take into account the results of all of these tests in conjunction with the patient's medical history.

WAYS HEPATITIS B CAN BE TRANSMITTED

Hepatitis B can spread in a variety of ways. Preventing the virus's spread necessitates an understanding of its modes of transmission. The most common routes by which hepatitis B can spread are as follows:

<u>Sexual Activity:</u> Unprotected sexual contact with an infected person can transmit hepatitis B. This incorporates vaginal, butt-centric, and oral sex. Mucous membranes or tiny skin cuts or tears can let the virus into the body.

<u>Blood-on-Blood Contact:</u> By coming into direct contact with infected blood, hepatitis B can be spread. This can happen when you share infected blood-contaminated needles, syringes, or other drug paraphernalia. Accidental needle stick injuries in healthcare facilities or other situations involving blood-to-blood contact can also result in this condition.

<u>Transmission from Mother to Child</u>: During labor, infected women can spread the virus to their unborn children. If the baby's open cuts or mucous membranes come into contact with the mother's blood or other infected fluids, the infection can spread. If the mother has cracked or bleeding nipples, breastfeeding can also spread hepatitis B.

<u>Utilization of Medical Equipment Contaminated:</u> Utilization of contaminated or improperly sterilized medical equipment can result in the transmission of hepatitis B. Needles, syringes, surgical instruments, tattooing, body piercing, and acupuncture tools are all examples of this.

<u>Sharing Private Things</u>: Hepatitis B transmission can result from sharing personal items that could come into contact with blood or other body fluids. Razors, toothbrushes, nail clippers, and any other item that might have traces of infected blood are examples of these items.

<u>Workplace Exposition:</u> Accidental needle stick injuries or direct contact with infected blood or body fluids may put healthcare providers or laboratory workers at risk for hepatitis B infection.

It is essential to keep in mind that neither respiratory droplets like coughing or sneezing nor casual contact like hugging, shaking hands, and sharing food or water transmit hepatitis B. For the virus to spread, it must be near infected blood, sperm, vaginal fluids, or other body fluids.

Vaccination is the most effective method of preventing infection, and prevention is essential to halting the spread of hepatitis B. Safe sex, barrier methods like condoms, and avoiding sharing personal items like needles can also help lower the risk of transmission. In healthcare settings, infection control practices must be followed to avoid occupational exposure.

PREVENTION OF HEPATITIS B

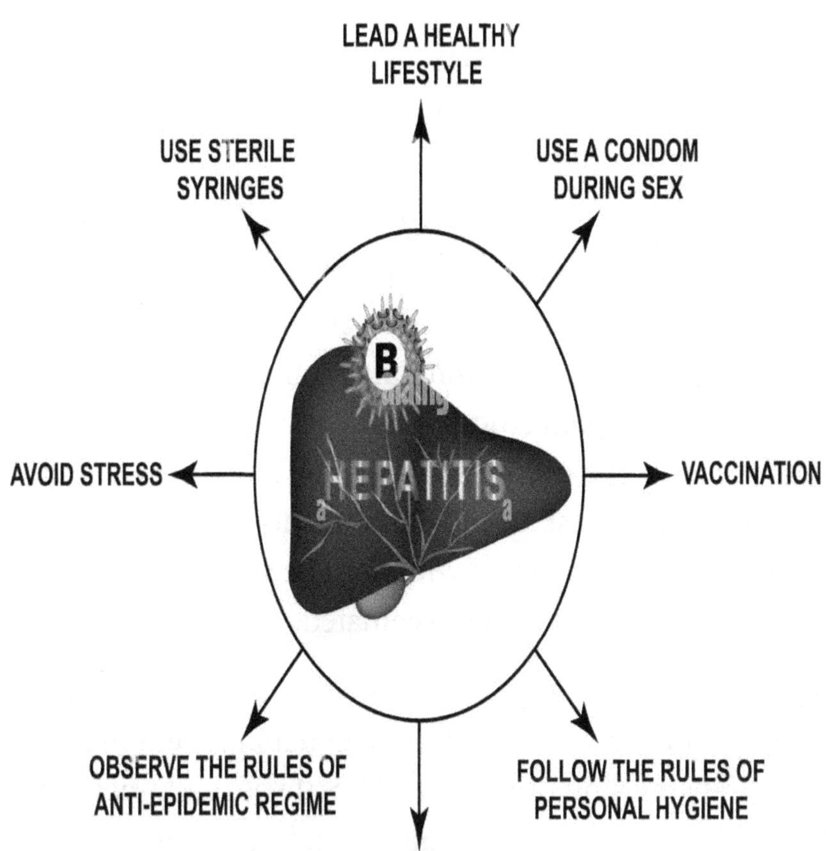

CHAPTER TWO
PREVENTION STRATEGIES

In order to cut down on the spread of hepatitis B, prevention strategies are essential. The following are specific steps you can take to lower your chances of getting the virus and spreading it:

Vaccination: Preventing hepatitis B infection is made extremely easy with the hepatitis B vaccine. Depending on the vaccine, it is given in a series of three or four doses. As part of routine immunization programs, the World Health Organization (WHO) recommends that all infants receive the hepatitis B vaccine. Adolescents and adults who are at risk of infection due to their occupation, lifestyle, or travel to areas with high hepatitis B prevalence should also get vaccinated.

Safe Sexual Behavior: Using barrier methods, such as condoms, during sexual activity can help prevent the sexual transmission of hepatitis B. Safe sexual practices include these practices. Although condom use does not provide complete protection, it does reduce the risk of transmission.

Reduced Risk Measures: People who inject drugs are less likely to spread hepatitis B if they don't share needles, syringes, or any other drug paraphernalia. Sterile injecting equipment, syringe exchange programs, and drug rehabilitation services can all help prevent infection.

<u>Preventing Transmission from Mother to Child</u>: All pregnant women should be tested for hepatitis B, and infants born to HBV-infected mothers should receive timely post-exposure prophylaxis, including the hepatitis B vaccine and hepatitis B immunoglobulin (HBIG) within 12 to 24 hours of birth. This is essential for reducing the long-term burden of hepatitis B. Culmination of the full hepatitis B immunization series is fundamental for long-haul assurance.

<u>Best Practices in Medicine</u>: To avoid occupational exposure and nosocomial transmission, it is essential to follow infection control procedures in healthcare settings. Utilizing single-use disposable needles and syringes, standard precautions like wearing gloves, masks, and protective clothing, and properly sterilizing medical equipment are all examples of this.

<u>Information and Awareness</u>: In order to lessen the stigma associated with the disease and encourage preventative actions, it is essential to raise awareness about hepatitis B, its modes of transmission, and methods of prevention. People can be empowered to protect themselves and make decisions based on accurate information through public health campaigns, educational programs in schools and communities, and other means.

Prevention and Early Treatment: Through screening programs, individuals infected with hepatitis B can be managed promptly and the risk of transmission is reduced. High-risk individuals, such as those who were born in areas with a high hepatitis B prevalence, individuals who have a history of injecting drugs, healthcare workers, and individuals who have multiple sexual partners, should undergo screening.

Care and Treatment: For people with chronic hepatitis B, having access to appropriate medical care, regular monitoring, and antiviral treatment can slow down viral replication, slow down liver damage, and lower the risk of complications. Preventing disease progression and improving long-term outcomes require prompt treatment start-up.

It is possible to reduce the prevalence and burden of hepatitis B and work toward its elimination as a public health threat by implementing these comprehensive prevention strategies.

THE IMPORTANCE OF HEPATITIS B VACCINATION

In order to prevent hepatitis B infection and its complications, hepatitis B vaccination is of the utmost importance. The following are the main reasons why getting vaccinated against hepatitis B is important:

<u>Highly Successful:</u> Preventing hepatitis B infection is made extremely easy with the hepatitis B vaccine. It provides immunity that lasts a long time and is more than 95% effective at preventing infection in adults and more than 90% effective at preventing chronic hepatitis B in infants and children.

<u>Chronic Infection Prevention:</u> Serious liver damage, cirrhosis, cancer of the liver, and even death are all possible outcomes of chronic hepatitis B infection. By stimulating the immune system to produce antibodies that are resistant to the virus, hepatitis B vaccination aids in the prevention of chronic infection. The vaccine significantly reduces the likelihood of long-term liver complications by preventing chronic infection.

<u>Guarding Against Liver Cancer:</u> Hepatocellular carcinoma (HCC), the most prevalent form of liver cancer, is primarily caused by chronic hepatitis B infection. Hepatitis B vaccination significantly reduces the incidence of liver cancer by preventing chronic infection. Vaccination during infancy has proven particularly effective in preventing liver cancer in later life and persistent infections.

Transmission Avoidance: Hepatitis B is a highly contagious virus that spreads easily through a variety of channels. In addition to safeguarding those who receive the vaccine, vaccination also contributes to the prevention of the virus's spread to others. The overall prevalence of hepatitis B can be decreased by achieving high vaccination coverage rates, resulting in a decrease in new infections.

Impact on the World: Millions of people around the world are affected by hepatitis B, which is a global health issue. Hepatitis B prevalence has been significantly reduced by vaccination programs in many nations. The number of new infections, chronic hepatitis B cases, and associated liver diseases has significantly decreased as a result of expanded vaccination efforts.

Cost-Effectiveness: In the long run, vaccination against hepatitis B has proven to be cost-effective. Vaccination reduces the need for costly medical interventions like antiviral treatments, liver transplants, and cancer therapies by preventing chronic infection and its complications, such as liver cirrhosis and cancer. Not only does this save lives, but it also lowers the cost of healthcare and benefits society as a whole.

Equity and universal coverage: The World Health Organization (WHO) recommends hepatitis B vaccination as part of routine childhood immunization programs. Equity in healthcare can be ensured by providing vaccinations to all, regardless of socioeconomic status. To further reduce health disparities, vaccination programs target vulnerable populations like infants, healthcare workers, people who inject drugs, and people who have multiple sexual partners.

In conclusion, getting vaccinated against hepatitis B is a safe, highly effective, and low-cost way to protect against the virus, chronic liver disease, and liver cancer. We can make significant progress toward eliminating hepatitis B as a public health threat and enhancing global health outcomes by vaccinating individuals, particularly during childhood.

CHRONIC HEPATITIS B
TRANSITION FROM ACUTE TO CHRONIC HEPATITIS B INFECTION AND THE LONG-TERM CONSEQUENCES

When the immune system is unable to eliminate the hepatitis B virus (HBV) from the body within six months of the initial infection, the condition moves from acute to chronic. Infants and young children are more likely to develop chronic infections, but adults who contract acute hepatitis B generally recover completely. For managing and preventing complications associated with chronic hepatitis B, it is essential to comprehend this transition and its long-term effects. The initial infection phase of acute hepatitis B typically lasts up to six months. People may experience fatigue, abdominal pain, jaundice, and flu-like symptoms during this phase. The virus is detected by the immune system, which launches an immune response to control and eliminate it. Most of the time, the immune system works to get rid of the infection, and people fully recover and become immune to future hepatitis B infections.

Chronic Infection with Hepatitis B: Chronic hepatitis B infection can result when the immune system is unable to eradicate the virus. Persistent disease is characterized as the steadiness of hepatitis B surface antigen (HBsAg) in the blood for over a half year. Laboratory markers and the degree of liver inflammation and fibrosis can divide chronic hepatitis B into distinct phases.

Long-Term Repercussions: Long-term effects of chronic hepatitis B infection include the following:

(A) Cirrhosis of the liver: Liver cirrhosis can develop as a result of chronic hepatitis B inflammation that persists for an extended period of time. Continuous liver damage and scarring that impairs liver function leads to cirrhosis. Ascites, or fluid accumulation in the abdomen, portal hypertension, liver failure, and an increased risk of liver cancer are all potential outcomes.

(B). Liver Cancer: Hepatocellular carcinoma the most common form of liver cancer, hepatocellular carcinoma (HCC), is more common in people who have had chronic hepatitis B infection. HCC develops as a result of ongoing inflammation in the liver and the incorporation of HBV DNA into liver cells. Through surveillance programs, regular monitoring and early detection can improve outcomes for people at risk.

(C). Manifestations beyond the liver: Various extra hepatic manifestations, or conditions that affect organs outside the liver, are linked to chronic hepatitis B infection. These include blood-related disorders, immune-mediated disorders like polyarthritis nodosa, kidney diseases like membranous nephropathy, and so on.

TREATMENT AND MANAGEMENT

Monitoring of liver function, viral load, and serological markers on a regular basis is necessary for managing chronic hepatitis B. Based on the risk of disease progression, the degree of liver inflammation, and viral replication, antiviral therapy may be prescribed. Antiviral medications can slow down the progression of liver disease, reduce inflammation, and suppress viral replication. In order to catch HCCs in their earliest stages and treat them, regular screenings for liver cancer are essential.

Vaccination is essential for preventing the spread of hepatitis B and reducing the likelihood of chronic infection and its long-term effects. Chronic hepatitis B can be reduced, improved outcomes can be achieved, and complications can be avoided with prompt identification, regular monitoring, and appropriate medical treatment.

HOW CHRONIC HEPATITIS B CAN LEAD TO LIVER CIRRHOSIS, LIVER FAILURE, AND LIVER CANCER

Multiple complications, including liver cirrhosis, liver failure, and liver cancer, can result from chronic hepatitis B infection. Each of these conditions can develop in the following ways:

<u>Liver Cirrhosis:</u> A progressive condition known as liver cirrhosis is characterized by the scarring of healthy liver tissue. Continuous inflammation in the liver causes a healing response in chronic hepatitis B infection, resulting in the accumulation of fibrous tissue over time. Scar tissue is formed as a result of this ongoing liver damage and repair process.

The liver's normal structure is disrupted by scar tissue, affecting its function. The liver becomes increasingly hard and nodular as cirrhosis progresses, making it less able to perform essential functions like filtering toxins, making proteins, storing vitamins, and making bile.

Ascites, which is a buildup of fluid in the abdomen, esophageal varices, which are enlarged blood vessels in the esophagus, and hepatic encephalopathy, which is brain dysfunction brought on by liver failure, are all complications of liver cirrhosis.

Failed Liver: In the end, chronic hepatitis B infection can lead to liver failure, in which the liver is severely damaged and unable to perform its essential functions. The liver's capacity for regeneration and proper function decreases as cirrhosis progresses.

Acute (sudden onset) or chronic (developing over time) forms of liver failure exist. Jaundice, which is a yellowing of the skin and eyes, abdominal pain, fatigue, nausea, vomiting, confusion, and bleeding disorders are all signs of liver failure. A liver transplant is frequently required in cases of acute liver failure, which is a medical emergency that requires immediate medical attention. To maintain the highest level of quality of life possible in patients with chronic liver failure, ongoing management and supportive care are essential.

Hepatocellular Carcinoma of the Liver: Hepatocellular carcinoma (HCC), the most common form of liver cancer, is significantly more likely to occur in people who have had chronic hepatitis B infection. Multiple factors contribute to the development of HCC in chronic hepatitis B:

(A) Constant inflammation of the liver: Cellular damage and regeneration are sparked by the hepatitis B virus's persistent inflammation in the liver. Genetic mutations that encourage the growth of cancer cells may result from this cycle of inflammation and regeneration.

(B) Integration of Viruses: The hepatitis B virus can sometimes incorporate its own DNA into the DNA of liver cell DNA. The liver cells' normal function is disrupted as a result of this integration, which may also contribute to the development of HCC.

(C) Cholangitis: Chronic hepatitis B can lead to liver cirrhosis, which significantly raises the risk of HCC. The cirrhosis-associated scar tissue and regenerative processes create an environment that encourages the growth of cancer cells.

For the early detection of liver cancer in people with chronic hepatitis B, regular surveillance with ultrasound and alpha-fetoprotein (AFP) blood tests is essential. This allows for prompt intervention, including curative treatment options like liver transplantation or localized ablation therapies.

To reduce the likelihood of these complications, it is essential to appropriately manage chronic hepatitis B infection. The progression of liver disease can be slowed down and long-term outcomes can be improved with timely interventions, medical advice, and regular monitoring. Vaccination against hepatitis B significantly lowers the risk of developing these severe liver-related complications and prevents chronic infection.

MONITORING AND MANAGING CHRONIC INFECTION, INCLUDING REGULAR CHECK-UPS, LIVER FUNCTION TESTS, AND ANTIVIRAL TREATMENT OPTIONS.

Regular checkups, liver function tests, and, if necessary, antiviral treatment are all necessary for managing chronic hepatitis B infection. The most important aspects of management and monitoring are as follows:

<u>Regular Examinations:</u> Patients with chronic hepatitis B should go to a doctor who knows how to treat liver diseases on a regular basis. The stage of liver disease, viral replication level, and presence of liver cirrhosis all have an impact on the frequency of checkups. In most cases, checkups should be done every six months to a year.

<u>Tests of Liver Function:</u> Blood tests called liver function tests are used to evaluate the liver's health and function. Various blood enzymes, proteins, and substances that indicate liver function, inflammation, and damage are measured in these tests. Common tests for liver function include:

a. Alanine aminotransferase (ALT) and aspartate aminotransferase (AST): Raised degrees of ALT and AST might show liver aggravation and harm.

b. Hemoglobin: The presence of liver dysfunction or a clog in the bile ducts can be indicated by elevated bilirubin levels.

c. Time for albumin and prothrombin: These tests look at how well the liver makes synthetic hormones and how well blood can clot.

d. Alpha-fetoprotein Hepatocellular carcinoma (liver cancer) can be monitored using AFP, a tumor marker.

The progression of the disease can be tracked, treatment response can be evaluated, and any signs of liver damage or complications can be identified by regularly monitoring liver function tests.

<u>**Testing for Viral Load**</u>: The amount of hepatitis B virus (HBV) in the blood is determined by viral load testing. It assists in monitoring the efficacy of antiviral treatment and determining the level of viral replication. While a high viral load may necessitate treatment or closer monitoring, a low viral load indicates a lower risk of disease progression.

<u>Imaging the Liver</u>: In order to evaluate the structure of the liver, spot signs of cirrhosis, and check for liver cancer, periodic liver imaging, such as an ultrasound or a computed tomography (CT) scan, may be recommended. Any nodules or abnormalities that might necessitate additional testing or treatment can be seen with imaging.

<u>Evaluation of Fibrosis:</u> The severity of liver damage and the likelihood of disease progression depend on the evaluation of liver fibrosis, or scarring. Without requiring a liver biopsy, non-invasive techniques like transient elastography (Fibro Scan) or blood-based fibrosis markers can estimate liver fibrosis.

<u>Treatment for the virus:</u> Various factors, such as the degree of liver inflammation, viral load, presence of liver cirrhosis, and risk of disease progression, may suggest antiviral treatment for chronic hepatitis B. Nucleos (t) ide analogs, such as entecavir and tenofovir, are antiviral medications that can slow down the progression of liver disease, reduce inflammation in the liver, and suppress viral replication.

The response to therapy and individual factors influence the length of antiviral treatment. In some cases, treatment may last a lifetime, while in others, a specific amount of time spent in therapy and close monitoring may be sufficient.

Surveillance of Hepatocellular Carcinoma:

Hepatocellular carcinoma (HCC) is more likely to occur in those with advanced liver disease or cirrhosis who have chronic hepatitis B. AFP levels and periodic imaging (ultrasound, CT scan, or MRI) are part of regular HCC surveillance. Individual risk factors and regional guidelines determine surveillance intervals.

Lifestyle adjustments: Changing one's lifestyle can support liver health and lower the likelihood of liver disease progressing. These include keeping a healthy weight, not drinking too much alcohol, having safe sex, not sharing needles or other drug paraphernalia, and getting the vaccines that are recommended (for hepatitis A and hepatitis B, for instance).

To effectively manage a chronic hepatitis B infection, regular monitoring, treatment adherence, and a healthy lifestyle are necessary. The proper management of chronic hepatitis B is ensured and the risk of complications is reduced through collaboration with a liver specialist.

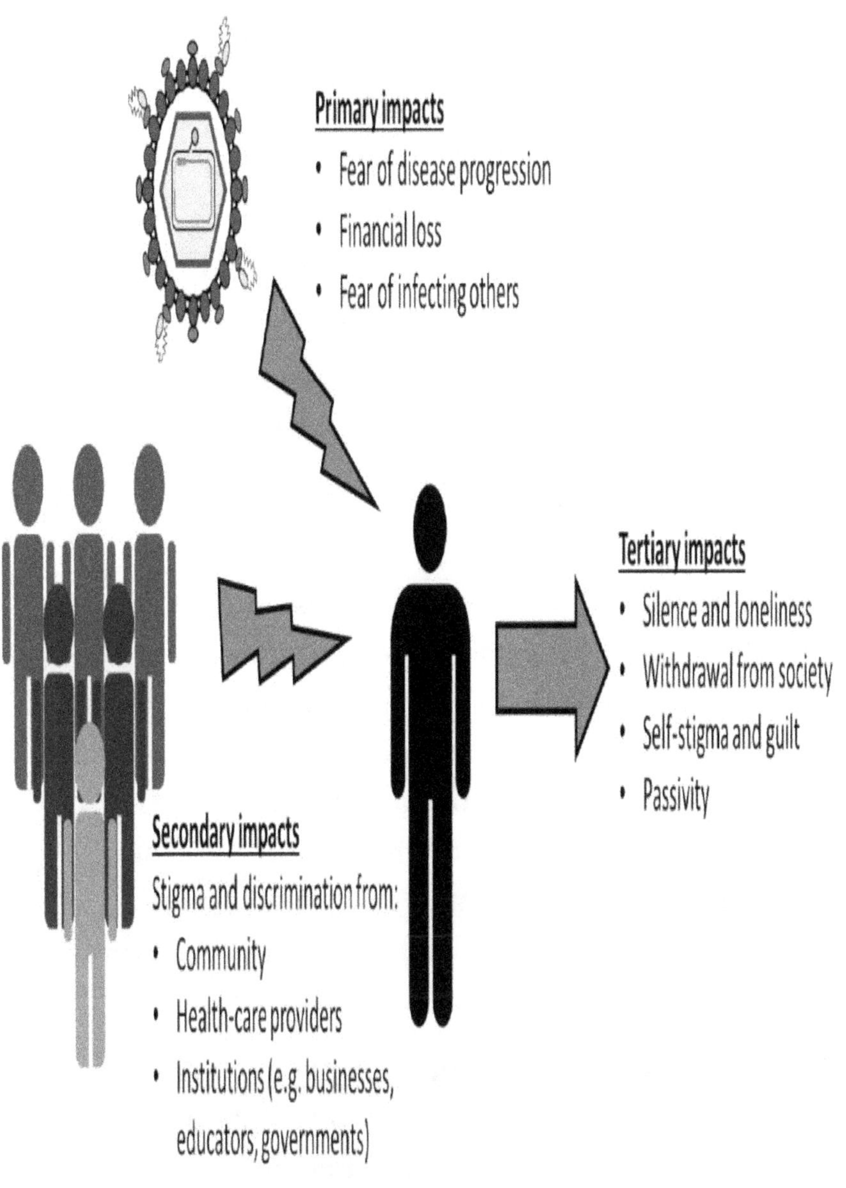

Primary impacts
• Fear of disease progression
• Financial loss
• Fear of infecting others

Tertiary impacts
• Silence and loneliness
• Withdrawal from society
• Self-stigma and guilt
• Passivity

Secondary impacts
Stigma and discrimination from:
• Community
• Health-care providers
• Institutions (e.g. businesses, educators, governments)

CHAPTER THREE
STIGMA AND DISCRIMINATION
SOCIAL STIGMA ASSOCIATED WITH HEPATITIS B AND THE IMPACT IT HAS ON INDIVIDUALS AND COMMUNITIES.

It is essential to address the hepatitis B social stigma because it has a significant impact on individuals and communities affected by the disease. An overview of the effects of and social stigma associated with hepatitis B is as follows:

Disparity and stigma: Hepatitis B is much of the time joined by friendly disgrace, which includes negative perspectives, convictions, and generalizations toward people living with the contamination. In the workplace, education, housing, relationships, and access to healthcare, stigma can result in discrimination and prejudice. Misunderstandings and apprehension regarding the disease can lead to exclusion, isolation, and unfair treatment for those with hepatitis B.

Misconceptions and a lack of awareness: A lack of awareness and misconceptions about hepatitis B frequently lead to stigma. A lot of people have false beliefs about how the disease spreads, associating it with high-risk behaviors or moral judgments. These misconceptions contribute to the stigmatization of hepatitis B sufferers, resulting in social barriers and the persistence of stigma in communities.

Effect on mental health: People with hepatitis B who are stigmatized may experience feelings of shame, guilt, embarrassment, and low self-esteem. These feelings can have severe psychological and emotional repercussions. They might also experience social withdrawal, anxiety, and depression, which can lower their quality of life and make them reluctant to get the help and care they need.

Effects on Testing and Disclosure: People who have hepatitis B may be reluctant to tell others about their infection status, including potential partners, employers, and healthcare providers. Individuals may be unable to obtain the necessary medical care, including testing, treatment, and preventative measures, because they are afraid of being judged or discriminated against. The virus may continue to spread within communities due to a lack of testing and disclosure.

Cultural and Community Factors: Cultural norms and beliefs can have an impact on hepatitis B stigma. In some cultures, infectious diseases like hepatitis B may carry a particularly negative stigma. A lack of education, cultural perceptions, and misconceptions can exacerbate stigma and impede effective disease management.

<u>Education and advocacy:</u> The social stigma of hepatitis B must be addressed through coordinated efforts to raise awareness, educate, and advocate. It is essential to dispel myths, disseminate accurate information regarding transmission and prevention, and stress that hepatitis B is a medical condition and not a reflection of a person's character or behavior. Stigma can be reduced and inclusion can be made more inclusive through targeted educational programs, community involvement, and public health campaigns.

<u>Education by peers and support networks</u>: People living with hepatitis B can feel empowered by creating support networks and participating in peer education programs. Connecting with others who have gone through something similar can help break up the isolation, provide emotional support, and encourage sharing of knowledge. Peer educators who have been personally affected by hepatitis B can be of great assistance in dispelling misconceptions, providing support, and combating stigma in their communities.

<u>Legal and Policy Protection:</u> The stigma and discrimination associated with hepatitis B can be reduced by policy measures. Equal rights and opportunities for people with hepatitis B can be ensured through legal protections against discrimination in employment, education, healthcare, and housing. However, it is essential to develop policies that prioritize equal access to healthcare, testing, treatment, and support services.

The social stigma of hepatitis B necessitates a multifaceted strategy that incorporates community involvement, advocacy, education, awareness, and policy changes. We can create a supportive environment for people who live with hepatitis B and work toward removing the barriers and prejudices they face by encouraging empathy, understanding, and inclusion.

THE IMPORTANCE OF DESTIGMATIZATION EFFORTS AND PROMOTING A SUPPORTIVE AND INCLUSIVE ENVIRONMENT FOR PEOPLE LIVING WITH HEPATITIS B

There are a number of reasons why DE stigmatization efforts and the creation of a welcoming and inclusive environment for those living with hepatitis B are necessary:

<u>Giving Individuals Power:</u> People with hepatitis B feel less shame, guilt, and isolation when they are DE stigmatized, giving them more power. They are able to openly talk about their condition, get the right medical care, and make well-informed decisions about their health thanks to this.

<u>Promoting Diagnostics and Testing:</u> Testing and diagnosis can be significantly impeded by stigma. By making hepatitis B less of a stigma, we make it easier for people to get tested and diagnosed without worrying about being judged or treated differently. For prompt medical intervention, treatment start-up, and transmission prevention, early diagnosis is essential.

<u>Promoting Healthcare Access</u>: People who are stigmatized may be less likely to seek medical care, which can result in inadequate treatment for their condition. We make it easier for people with hepatitis B to get healthcare by creating a supportive environment. This makes it possible for people with hepatitis B to get regular checks, monitors, and the right medical care to effectively manage their condition.

<u>To Avoid Transmission:</u> Conversations about hepatitis B, transmission routes, and prevention measures are more likely to take place in an environment that is welcoming and supportive. This information enables individuals to take proactive measures to safeguard their loved ones and prevent transmission. DE stigmatization efforts help raise awareness and encourage safer behaviors like not sharing needles, getting vaccinated, and having safe sex.

<u>Increasing Well-Being and Mental Health</u>: Mental health can be negatively affected by hepatitis B stigma, which can cause anxiety, depression, and social isolation.

We prioritize the mental health and well-being of people with hepatitis B by creating an inclusive and supportive environment, improving their overall quality of life.

<u>Promoting Awareness and Education</u>: DE stigmatization efforts involve educating communities, healthcare providers, and the general public about hepatitis B. We make a contribution to a society that is better informed and more empathetic by dispelling myths, providing accurate information, and raising awareness. This information enables people to challenge trashing perspectives and ways of behaving.

<u>Promoting Support and Advocacy:</u> Support groups, peer networks, and organizations dedicated to hepatitis B provide a platform for sharing experiences, providing emotional support, and advocating for improved policies and services. DE stigmatization efforts encourage advocacy for the rights and needs of individuals living with hepatitis B.

<u>Promoting Social Justice and Equity</u>: Equity and social justice are reflected in the treatment of hepatitis B stigma. It ensures that people with hepatitis B have equal access to opportunities, healthcare, employment, education, and social participation without bias or discrimination.

Individuals, communities, healthcare providers, policymakers, and advocacy organizations all need to work together on DE stigmatization efforts. We can create a society that embraces and supports people who live with hepatitis B, thereby lessening the impact of stigma and improving their overall well-being. We can do this by promoting education, awareness, empathy, and inclusivity.

TREATMENT AND CARE
AVAILABLE TREATMENT OPTIONS FOR HEPATITIS B

The goals of the various treatments for chronic hepatitis B are to stop the spread of the virus, lessen inflammation in the liver, and stop the disease from getting worse. The use of antiviral medications is the main treatment strategy. An overview of the treatments that are available, as well as their potential benefits and drawbacks:

<u>Antiviral Treatments:</u>

a. Analogues of nucleotides (NAs): Antiviral therapy for chronic hepatitis B typically consists primarily of nucleos (t) ide analogs, such as entecavir, *tenofovir disoproxil fumarate (TDF), (TAF), lamivudine, adefovir, and telbivudine*. By reducing the body's overall viral load and inhibiting viral replication, these medications work.

b. Advantages: The hepatitis B virus can be controlled, liver damage can be avoided, and the progression of the disease can be slowed down by taking antiviral medications. They can lower the risk of complications like cirrhosis and liver cancer, improve liver function, and reduce inflammation in the liver. The long-term suppression of the virus that is offered by antiviral treatment also has the potential to improve overall health outcomes.

c. Possible Negative Effects: Depending on the drug, antiviral medications can cause side effects. Although the majority of NAs are generally well tolerated, potential side effects include muscle or joint pain, nausea, diarrhea, and fatigue. Rarely, severe side effects like toxicity to the kidneys or liver may occur. While receiving antiviral treatment, regular monitoring and discussing potential side effects with a healthcare provider are essential.

Interferon-alpha pegylated (Peg-IFN): An alternative treatment for chronic hepatitis B is pegylated interferon-alpha, which is given as an injection and boosts the body's immune response to the virus.

a. Advantages: In some people, Peg-IFN can assist in maintaining viral suppression, increasing the likelihood of long-term remission. It has the advantage of having a set amount of time to treat (typically 48 weeks) and the possibility of a long-lasting treatment response even after stopping treatment.

b. Possible Negative Effects: Treatment with peg-IFN can lead to depression and flu-like symptoms like fatigue, fever, and muscle aches. Reactions at the injection site, changes in mood, thyroid dysfunction, and hematological abnormalities are additional potential side effects. Peg-IFN should not be taken by people with advanced liver disease or cirrhosis because there is a possibility that liver function will get worse.

<u>Combinational Treatment:</u> To improve treatment response, a combination of NA and Peg-IFN therapy may be considered in some instances. However, combination therapy is not widely used as a standard treatment because it requires careful evaluation.

The stage of liver disease, viral load, liver function, the presence of cirrhosis, and individual patient factors all influence the choice of treatment. The selection of the most effective treatment option can be guided by healthcare providers who have experience managing hepatitis B.

It is essential to keep in mind that although antiviral medications have the ability to effectively control viral replication, they may not completely eradicate the hepatitis B virus from the body. In this way, standard checking, adherence to treatment, and long haul the board are fundamental for ideal results.

In order to make well-informed decisions regarding their hepatitis B treatment plan, individuals who are considering or are currently receiving treatment ought to talk to their healthcare provider about the advantages, potential side effects, and requirements for monitoring.

IMPORTANCE OF HEALTHCARE PROVIDER INVOLVEMENT IN MANAGING THE DISEASE AND SUPPORTING PATIENTS.

In managing hepatitis B and supporting patients throughout their disease journey, healthcare provider involvement is essential. The following are some important reasons why healthcare providers are so important:

<u>Accurate Monitoring and Diagnosis:</u> Various blood tests and assessments are used to accurately diagnose hepatitis B by healthcare professionals. They are able to assess liver function, track the progression of the disease, and determine the stage of the infection. Healthcare professionals are able to monitor changes in viral load, liver enzymes, and liver health through regular monitoring, which enables prompt interventions when they are required.

<u>Guidance for Treatment</u>: Because they are well-versed in the various treatment options for hepatitis B, healthcare professionals are able to help patients comprehend the advantages, potential drawbacks, and long-term effects of various treatment options. Healthcare professionals are able to tailor treatment plans to each patient's specific requirements by taking into account individual patient factors like liver function, the stage of liver disease, and comorbidities.

<u>Management of Antiviral Treatment</u>: A key component of managing chronic hepatitis B is antiviral therapy. Antiviral treatment is initiated, monitored, and adjusted by healthcare providers based on the patient's response to therapy. They regularly monitor the viral load, liver enzymes, and other relevant biomarkers to determine the efficacy of the treatment.

<u>Preventative Actions:</u> To safeguard patients and prevent transmission to others, healthcare providers emphasize the significance of preventative measures. They instruct patients on safe sex rehearses, the requirement for hepatitis B immunization for them and close contacts, and precautionary measures to forestall sharing of needles or other likely wellsprings of viral transmission.

<u>Managing Comorbidities and Co-Infections:</u> Hepatitis B and other infections, like HIV or hepatitis C, can coexist. Medical services suppliers assist with dealing with these co-diseases and give extensive consideration. They also address comorbidities like diabetes, cardiovascular disease, and complications related to the liver, all of which may necessitate additional treatment strategies.

Counseling and education: Patients and their families can benefit greatly from the education and counseling provided by healthcare providers. They talk about the nature of hepatitis B, how it spreads, and how to prevent it. They also address any misconceptions, fears, or attitudes that put the disease in a negative light. Patients are empowered by healthcare providers to make well-informed decisions regarding their health and well-being by receiving accurate information.

Patient Advocacy and Emotional Support: The stigma, anxiety, and uncertainty surrounding the progression of hepatitis B can make living with the disease emotionally taxing. Patients receive emotional support from healthcare professionals, who address their concerns and offer direction throughout the journey. As patient advocates, they ensure that patients' rights are upheld and that healthcare systems treat them with compassion, understanding, and respect.

Collaboration and Recommendations: Patients can be referred to hepatologists, gastroenterologists, or other specialists with experience managing liver diseases when they require specialized care or interventions. In addition, they collaborate with counselors, social workers, and support groups in order to provide comprehensive patient care and support.

For patients with hepatitis B to receive comprehensive support, effective disease management, and improved treatment outcomes, healthcare providers must be involved. Their expertise, direction, and compassionate care are crucial to enhancing the patients' overall well-being.

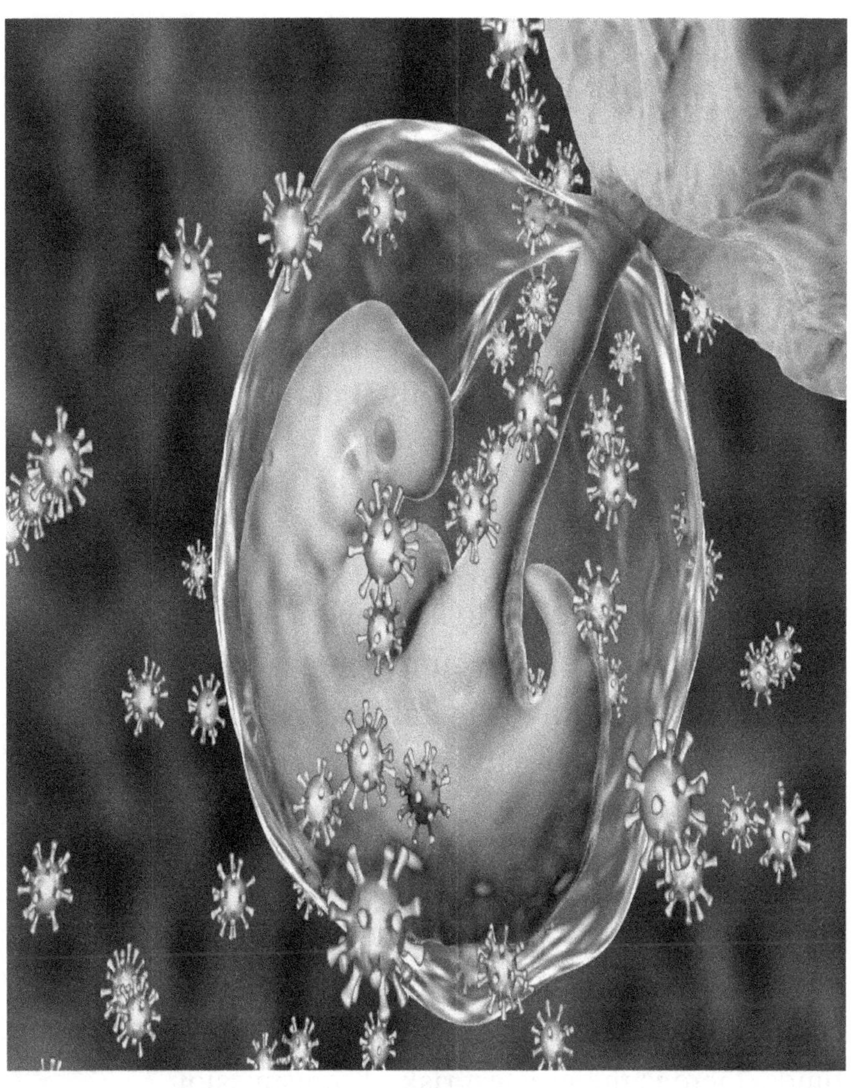

CHAPTER FOUR
HEPATITIS B AND PREGNANCY
CONCERNS AND CONSIDERATIONS RELATED TO HEPATITIS B DURING PREGNANCY

For people who have hepatitis B, pregnancy brings with it a unique set of worries and considerations. The most important points about hepatitis B during pregnancy are as follows:

Transmission from above: The risk of vertical transmission, or the transmission of the hepatitis B virus from an infected mother to her unborn child, is the primary cause of concern during pregnancy. For infants born to mothers with high viral loads, the risk of vertical transmission without intervention can range anywhere from 70% to 90%.

Transmission Timing: During pregnancy, childbirth, or the postpartum period through breastfeeding, vertical transmission can occur. During labor, when the baby comes into contact with the mother's blood and bodily fluids, there is the greatest risk of transmission.

Preventative Actions: Implementing preventive measures, such as the following, is essential to preventing vertical transmission:

a. Treatment for the virus: Pregnant women with high viral loads (viral load >200,000 IU/mL) during the third trimester of pregnancy may be prescribed antiviral medications, specifically Tenofovir disoproxil fumarate (TDF). By halting viral replication, antiviral treatment significantly lowers the likelihood of vertical transmission.

b. Hepatitis B Immunization: The hepatitis B vaccine should be given to every newborn within 24 hours of their birth. The risk of vertical transmission is further reduced when this vaccination and hepatitis B immunoglobulin (HBIG) are given to infants born to mothers with a high viral load.

<u>Monitoring and Reporting:</u> During pregnancy, pregnant women with hepatitis B should have their viral load, liver function, and overall health checked on a regular basis. This observing assists medical services suppliers with deciding the suitable timing and span of antiviral therapy, if essential.

<u>Considerations for Delivery</u>: The choice of delivery method for pregnant women with hepatitis B—vaginal delivery or cesarean section—is up for debate. Unless there are additional reasons to use this method of delivery, a cesarean section is not typically recommended solely to prevent vertical transmission of hepatitis B.

<u>Considerations for Breastfeeding:</u> The mother's viral load, the baby's hepatitis B vaccination status, and other considerations should all be taken into account when making a decision about breastfeeding. If the newborn has received the hepatitis B vaccine and HBIG shortly after birth, breastfeeding is generally considered safe.

<u>Monitoring after delivery:</u> After birth, infants born to mothers infected with hepatitis B should be closely monitored. Following the recommended course of the hepatitis B vaccine, they should have antibody testing to verify their immunity. In order to check for any signs of hepatitis B infection and ensure the baby's health, regular follow-up visits are essential.

<u>Education and Support:</u> Healthcare providers should provide pregnant women with hepatitis B with comprehensive support and education. Counseling on preventative measures, treatment options, potential dangers, and the significance of adhering to medical recommendations are all part of this. It is essential to address any concerns, offer emotional support, and connect people with the appropriate support networks and resources.

Individualized treatment plans for pregnant people with hepatitis B must be developed in close collaboration with their healthcare providers and take into account their particular circumstances. The risk of vertical transmission can be significantly reduced through preventative measures and medical interventions, safeguarding the mother's and baby's health and well-being.

TRANSMISSION RISKS, PREVENTIVE MEASURES, AND THE IMPORTANCE OF PRENATAL SCREENING AND VACCINATION.

RISKS OF TRANSMISSION: Hepatitis B can spread in several ways, including:

<u>Vertical Transmission:</u> During childbirth, an infected mother transmits the virus to her unborn child. Vertical transmission carries a high risk if preventative measures are not taken.

<u>Body Fluids and Blood:</u> Direct contact with infected blood or body fluids can spread hepatitis B. Sharing personal items like toothbrushes or razors, unprotected sexual contact, accidental needle stick injuries, or sharing needles or other drug paraphernalia is all examples of this.

<u>Workplace Exposition:</u> If proper infection control measures are not followed, healthcare workers and others who are at risk of being exposed to blood and body fluids are at risk for hepatitis B transmission.

<u>Unhealthy Medical Procedures:</u> Hepatitis B can be spread by contaminated medical instruments like needles, syringes, and surgical equipment in settings with poor infection control practices.

PREVENTATIVE ACTIONS:

<u>Vaccination:</u> Hepatitis B immunization is the best preventive measure. The vaccine is recommended for all infants, children, adolescents, and adults because it is safe and very effective. To achieve long-term immunity, the vaccine requires multiple doses.

<u>Prenatal Examination:</u> To identify infected mothers and take appropriate preventative measures, prenatal hepatitis B screening is essential. Testing for hepatitis B surface antigen (HBsAg) typically occurs during the first prenatal visit or early pregnancy.

<u>Immunoglobulin for hepatitis B (HBIG):</u> Along with the hepatitis B vaccine, infants born to mothers with high viral loads should receive HBIG within 12 to 24 hours of birth. Hepatitis B Vaccine for Newborns: HBIG provides immediate passive immunity against hepatitis B. All infants, no matter what the mother's hepatitis B status, ought to get the hepatitis B antibody somewhere around 24 hours after birth. To ensure long-term protection, the vaccine is given in multiple doses.

Techniques for Safe Injections: Medical services settings should stick to severe contamination control works, including the utilization of clean gear, legitimate removal of needles and sharps, and adherence to standard safeguards to forestall transmission through medical care techniques.

Safe Sexual Behavior: During sexual activity, the correct and consistent use of barrier methods like condoms can lower the risk of sexual transmission.

PRENATAL VACCINATION AND SCREENING ARE CRUCIAL:

Identifying Mothers Infected: Healthcare professionals can take the necessary preventative measures to lessen the likelihood of vertical transmission by identifying mothers with hepatitis B through prenatal screening.

Preventative Care: The risk of vertical transmission is significantly reduced by early intervention, such as antiviral treatment during pregnancy, made possible by prenatal screening.

Security for Babies: When given to newborns, the hepatitis B vaccine provides early protection against the virus, lowering the likelihood of infection and related complications.

<u>Breaking the Transmission Chain:</u> Breaking the chain of hepatitis B transmission from one generation to the next can only be accomplished through prenatal screening and vaccination. Over time, the overall prevalence of hepatitis B can be reduced by identifying the virus and preventing its transmission to newborns.

<u>Impact on Public Health</u>: By reducing the burden of hepatitis B and its associated complications, such as cirrhosis and liver cancer, prenatal screening, and vaccination programs contribute to public health efforts.

Comprehensive hepatitis B prevention strategies include prenatal screening and vaccination. We can significantly reduce the spread of hepatitis B and improve the overall health outcomes for mothers and infants by identifying infected individuals, providing timely interventions, and ensuring that newborns receive the necessary protection.

PREVALENCE OF HEPATITIS B WORLDWIDE

Hepatitis B is a major global health issue whose prevalence rates vary by region and population. An overview of the global prevalence of hepatitis B, with an emphasis on populations and regions at high risk:

<u>Prevalence Worldwide:</u> In 2019, the World Health Organization (WHO) estimated that 257 million people around the world were infected with chronic hepatitis B.

Africa, parts of Asia, and the Western Pacific, which includes countries like China and Vietnam, are where hepatitis B is most common.

High-Commonness Locales:

Africa, **a**. An estimated 6.1 percent of the population in Sub-Saharan Africa is infected with hepatitis B on a chronic basis, making it the region with the highest global prevalence. The low vaccination coverage, limited access to healthcare, and perinatal and early childhood transmission are all responsible for the high prevalence.

b. Asia: Hepatitis B is prevalent in a number of Asian nations; for instance, the prevalence can exceed 8% in Southeast Asian nations like Cambodia, Laos, and Vietnam. China and Mongolia likewise have critical hepatitis B loads.

c. Islands in the Pacific Hepatitis B is prevalent in many Pacific Island nations, including Papua New Guinea and some Pacific Island nations. In some areas, prevalence rates exceed 10%.

d. Areas in the Arctic Hepatitis B is more common in indigenous populations in the Arctic, including Alaska Native and Inuit populations, than in the general population.

Populations at High Risk:

a. Users of injected drugs (IDUs): Due to the sharing of contaminated needles and drug paraphernalia, IDUs are at a high risk of contracting hepatitis B.

b. MSM, or men who have sex with men: Due to exposure to other sexually transmitted diseases and unprotected sexual practices, MSM are more likely to contract hepatitis B.

c. Refugees and Migrants: Travelers from locales with high hepatitis B commonness might convey the disease, and evacuees might have restricted admittance to medical services and immunization.

d. Workers in Healthcare: Hepatitis B occupational exposure is possible for healthcare workers who come into contact with bodily fluids and blood. e. Infants born to infected mothers: Vertical transmission during childbirth is a possibility for infants born to mothers with chronic hepatitis B infection.

Economic and social factors: Hepatitis B is more common in some populations and regions due to socioeconomic factors like poverty, a lack of access to healthcare, poor sanitation and hygiene, and crowded living conditions.

Comprehensive prevention strategies, such as vaccination programs, increased awareness, accessibility to healthcare services, vertical transmission prevention, and targeted interventions for high-risk groups, are necessary to address the high prevalence of hepatitis B in these populations and regions.

It is essential to keep in mind that although hepatitis B is more prevalent in some populations and regions, the disease can affect individuals worldwide. For the prevention, management, and control of hepatitis B in all populations, screening, vaccination, and access to appropriate healthcare services are essential.

EFFORTS AND INITIATIVES UNDERTAKEN BY GOVERNMENTS, ORGANIZATIONS, AND COMMUNITIES TO CONTROL AND PREVENT THE SPREAD OF HEPATITIS B.

Worldwide, significant efforts have been made by governments, organizations, and communities to control and prevent the spread of hepatitis B. The following are some key initiatives and strategies that were implemented:

Programs for Vaccination: Numerous nations have implemented hepatitis B vaccination programs that target young children, adolescents, and high-risk populations. The goal of these programs is to lessen the spread of the virus and increase vaccination rates. Vaccination is frequently included in routine vaccination schedules or made available through specialized campaigns aimed at particular age groups or populations.

<u>Campaigns for Education and Awareness</u>: To raise awareness of hepatitis B, its modes of transmission, methods of prevention, and the significance of vaccination, governments, healthcare organizations, and community groups conduct awareness and education campaigns. To prevent transmission, these campaigns aim to reduce stigma, encourage early diagnosis, and encourage behavior change.

Testing and screening: Initiatives for hepatitis B screening and testing are promoted by governments and healthcare systems, with a focus on pregnant women and high-risk populations. Programs for screening aid in the identification of infected individuals who may require medical treatment or preventative measures. Outreach programs and free or discounted testing services for underserved populations may be part of testing campaigns.

<u>Vertical Transmission Avoidance</u>: The vertical transmission of hepatitis B from infected mothers to their unborn children is discouraged. Pregnant women should be screened regularly, antiviral medication should be given during pregnancy if necessary, newborns should be given the hepatitis B vaccine and hepatitis B immunoglobulin (HBIG), and breastfeeding advice should be based on individual risk assessments.

Safety for Healthcare Workers: To guarantee the safety of healthcare workers, both governments and healthcare organizations have implemented measures. These include procedures for reporting and managing occupational exposures, access to personal protective equipment, proper sharps handling and disposal, and infection control training.

Support for Populations at High Risk: High-risk groups like injecting drug users, MSM, migrants, and refugees are the focus of specific programs and interventions. Programs for reducing harm, accessibility to sterile needles and syringes, testing and connection to care, and culturally sensitive healthcare services are among these efforts.

Integrity with Health Care Systems: The integration of hepatitis B control and prevention measures into the larger health systems, including primary healthcare services, is a goal pursued by governments. This includes making sure that affordable antiviral medications are available and that hepatitis B testing, vaccination, and treatment are included in routine healthcare delivery.

<u>Collaboration on a global scale:</u> Countries with high hepatitis B prevalence collaborate with regional health agencies and partnerships, and international organizations like the World Health Organization (WHO), to develop guidelines, share best practices, provide technical assistance, and support capacity-building efforts. They coordinate efforts to address the global impact of hepatitis B and facilitate knowledge sharing. Community Engagement and Advocacy: Advocacy groups and community-based organizations play a crucial role in spreading awareness, providing assistance, and advocating for improved programs and policies. They work to end the stigma, give people who have hepatitis B more control over their lives, and get communities to help with prevention and control.

Vaccination, screening, education, healthcare system integration, and targeted interventions are just some of the many strategies needed to control and prevent hepatitis B. Joint effort among states, associations, medical services suppliers, and networks is fundamental to accomplish compelling avoidance and control of hepatitis B and diminish its weight on people and social orders.

AUTOIMMUNE HEPATITIS

The body's immune system mistakenly attacks healthy liver cells, resulting in inflammation and liver damage in autoimmune hepatitis, a chronic liver disease. Because the immune system, which is meant to protect the body from foreign substances like bacteria and viruses, instead targets the liver cells as if they were foreign, it is categorized as an autoimmune disorder.

The following are some important facts about autoimmune hepatitis:

Causes: It is unclear exactly what causes autoimmune hepatitis. It is thought to be the result of immune system deregulation, environmental triggers, and genetic predisposition all working together. The autoimmune response may be triggered by infections, drugs, and toxins, among other things, in susceptible people.

Types: Based on the antibodies that are present in the blood and the specific immune cells involved, autoimmune hepatitis is divided into two main types:

a. Autoimmune hepatitis of type 1: This is the most prevalent form, affecting between 80 and 90 percent of cases. It affects both sexes equally and can take place at any age. Specific autoantibodies, such as antinuclear antibodies (ANA) and smooth muscle antibodies (SMA), are linked to type 1 autoimmune hepatitis.

b. Autoimmune hepatitis of type 2: Type 2 autoimmune hepatitis is less prevalent and mostly affects young children. It is identified by the presence of autoantibodies known as anti-liver cytosol antibody type 1 (LC-1) and/or liver-kidney microsomal antibodies type 1 (LKM-1).

<u>Symptoms:</u> The signs and symptoms of autoimmune hepatitis can be mild or severe, and they can appear suddenly or gradually. Fatigue, abdominal pain or discomfort, jaundice (yellowing of the skin and eyes), dark urine, pale stools, loss of appetite, weight loss, and joint pain are all common symptoms. Some people can have no symptoms at first and be diagnosed through routine blood tests.

<u>Diagnosis:</u> A combination of clinical evaluation, blood tests, imaging studies, and a liver biopsy are used to make the diagnosis of autoimmune hepatitis. Liver inflammation, elevated liver enzymes, and the presence of particular autoantibodies are all possible outcomes of blood tests. Imaging tests like an MRI or ultrasound can be used to rule out other causes of liver disease and assess the health of the liver. Most of the time, a liver biopsy is done to confirm the diagnosis, figure out how bad the damage is to the liver, and decide what kind of treatment to give.

<u>Treatment:</u> The treatment of autoimmune hepatitis aims to reduce liver inflammation and suppress the abnormal immune response. Long-term administration of immunosuppressive medications like corticosteroids (like prednisone) and other immunosuppressant (like azathioprine) is the primary treatment. The autoimmune response can be controlled with these medications, preventing further liver damage. To maintain disease control and minimize side effects, medication doses must be monitored and adjusted frequently.

<u>Prognosis:</u> Most people with autoimmune hepatitis can go into remission and live normal lives with the right treatment and management. However, the disease can progress to advanced liver damage, cirrhosis, or even liver failure if it is not treated. Close observation, adherence to drugs, and normal development with medical care suppliers are urgent for long-haul executives and counteraction of entanglements.

A complicated and persistent liver disease, autoimmune hepatitis necessitates ongoing medical care and support. To manage their condition, maintain liver health, and monitor for any potential complications, people with autoimmune hepatitis need to collaborate closely with their healthcare providers.

HEPATITIS B COOKBOOK

Since there is no specific diet for hepatitis B, there is no "hepatitis B cookbook" available. However, a well-balanced and healthy diet can help people with hepatitis B maintain liver health and overall well-being. The following are some general dietary guidelines for people who have hepatitis B:

Proper nutrition: Hold back nothing adjusted diet that incorporates different natural products, vegetables, entire grains, lean proteins (like poultry, fish, vegetables, and tofu), and solid fats. Fiber, antioxidants, and essential nutrients can all be found in this to help the liver function.

Moderate intake of fat: Saturated and Tran's fats, in particular, should be limited in quantity. Reduce your intake of fried foods, processed snacks, and high-fat dairy products in favor of healthier fat sources like olive oil, nuts, seeds, and avocados.

Drink less: Because alcohol can exacerbate hepatitis B-related liver inflammation and cause additional liver damage, it is essential to avoid or limit alcohol consumption.

Hydration: To stay hydrated throughout the day, drink a lot of water. To support liver health, drink water, herbal teas, and other non-caffeinated beverages.

Moderation of sodium: To support liver health and reduce fluid retention, reduce sodium intake. Instead of relying on excessive salt, choose whole, fresh foods and flavor your meals with herbs, spices, and other flavorings.

<u>Individualized Changes:</u> It's important to remember that everyone has different dietary requirements. Dietary changes may be suggested based on the severity of liver damage and any associated health conditions. Consult a medical professional or a registered dietitian for individualized dietary advice tailored to your requirements.

You can look into general healthy cookbooks or recipe websites that focus on meals that are healthy and good for the liver, even though there may not be a specific hepatitis B cookbook available. Find recipes that follow the aforementioned guidelines, such as including a wide variety of vibrant fruits and vegetables, lean proteins, whole grains, and healthy fats. Your meals can be enjoyable and nutritious by experimenting with flavors and cooking methods.

To effectively manage hepatitis B, a healthy diet should be complemented by regular medical examinations, treatment adherence, and ongoing care from healthcare professionals.

HEPATITIS SUPPLEMENT

It is essential to note that I am not a healthcare professional but rather an AI language model. As a result, I am unable to give medical advice or recommend any particular supplements for hepatitis B. However, I can provide some general information regarding supplements and hepatitis B. When it comes to managing hepatitis B, it is necessary to place a priority on the medical treatments that have been prescribed to you and to follow the instructions given by medical professionals. Although they should not be used in place of medical treatment, supplements may contribute to better health as a whole. Consultation with a healthcare professional, such as a hepatologist or a registered dietitian, who can assess your specific condition and make tailored recommendations, is essential before taking supplements.

Consider these a few points:

<u>Nutrient and Mineral Enhancements</u>: There may be particular nutritional requirements for people who have chronic liver diseases like hepatitis B. Vitamins and minerals may be lacking in some instances. Through blood tests, a healthcare professional can determine whether you require any particular vitamin or mineral supplements.

<u>Dietary and herbal supplements</u>: There are a lot of herbal and dietary supplements out there that say they help the liver or the immune system. However, because their safety and efficacy are not always well-established or regulated, it is essential to exercise caution when using such supplements. Some herbal supplements can cause liver damage or interact with medications. Before taking any herbal or dietary supplements, it is essential to discuss this with your doctor.

Thistle of Milk: Milk thistle is a well-known herb that supports the liver frequently. It may have antioxidant and anti-inflammatory effects that may be beneficial to liver health, according to some studies. Nonetheless, more exploration is expected to lay out its viability explicitly for hepatitis B. Assuming you are thinking about milk thorn or some other natural enhancement, it is vital to examine it with your medical care supplier to decide on suitable doses, expected cooperation, and any possible dangers.

In conclusion, medical treatments for hepatitis B should not be substituted for supplements. You should talk to healthcare professionals who are familiar with your medical history and can give you specific advice. They can evaluate your particular nutritional requirements and guide the appropriateness, dosage, and safety of any supplements.

CONCLUSION
PERSONAL STORIES AND EXPERIENCES OF INDIVIDUALS LIVING WITH HEPATITIS B

The personal experiences and stories of people who have hepatitis B provide valuable insights into the difficulties they face, the successes they achieve, and the effects the disease has on their lives. These narratives all share a few recurring themes, which are as follows:

Initial Actions and Diagnosis: Numerous people share their encounters with getting a hepatitis B conclusion. When they found out about their condition, they say they were shocked, afraid, and confused. As they try to comprehend the disease's implications, the diagnosis frequently causes a period of uncertainty.

Disparity and stigma: Misconceptions about hepatitis B frequently result in stigma and discrimination against those who have the virus. Others, including friends, family, coworkers, and even healthcare professionals, may exhibit negative attitudes toward them. Social exclusion, strained relationships, and feelings of shame and self-blame are all possible outcomes of stigma.

Impact on Emotion and Psychology: Having hepatitis B can hurt one's mental and emotional health. They may experience feelings of anxiety, depression, and uncertainty regarding their future.. It can be emotionally challenging to be afraid of spreading the virus to loved ones or potential partners.

Effects on Family Dynamics and Relationships:
Relationships with intimate partners and family members can be impacted by hepatitis B. Fearing rejection or judgment, some people find it difficult to tell loved ones about their situation. Others face difficulties in starting a family or keeping close relationships while controlling the transmission risk.

Clinical Administration and Treatment: The challenges of adhering to long-term medication regimens, navigating potential side effects, and the requirement for regular monitoring and follow-up appointments are discussed in personal stories, which shed light on the experiences of individuals undergoing medical management and treatment for hepatitis B.

Empowerment and Protest: Stories of perseverance, empowerment, and advocacy are shared by many people with hepatitis B. They actively advocate for improved access to healthcare services, support networks, and resources, combat stigma, and raise awareness. They become advocates for change and gain strength by connecting with others in similar circumstances.

<u>Getting to Your Personal Goals:</u> Despite the difficulties, people with hepatitis B also celebrate their victories and accomplishments. They tell stories of accomplishments, happy relationships, and successful careers that show how resilient people are and how determined they are to live happy lives despite the disease.

RELIABLE RESOURCES, SUCH AS WEBSITES, ORGANIZATIONS, AND SUPPORT GROUPS, THAT OFFER ADDITIONAL INFORMATION, GUIDANCE, AND SUPPORT FOR INDIVIDUALS AFFECTED BY HEPATITIS B.

Certainly! Here is a list of reliable resources, websites, organizations, and support groups that provide valuable information, guidance, and support for individuals affected by hepatitis B:

<u>World Health Organization (WHO):</u> The WHO provides comprehensive information on hepatitis B, including global strategies, guidelines, and resources for prevention, diagnosis, and treatment. Their website offers fact sheets, publications, and updates on hepatitis B-related initiatives. Website: www.who.int/hepatitis/en/

<u>Centers for Disease Control and Prevention (CDC):</u> The CDC's website features extensive information on hepatitis B, including resources for healthcare professionals, guidelines for testing and vaccination, and educational materials for the general public. Website: www.cdc.gov/hepatitis/hbv/index.htm

<u>Hepatitis B Foundation:</u> The Hepatitis B Foundation is a non-profit organization dedicated to promoting hepatitis B research, advocacy, and support. Their website offers educational resources, fact sheets, clinical trial information, and support group directories. Website: www.hepb.org

<u>American Liver Foundation (ALF):</u> The ALF provides information on various liver diseases, including hepatitis B. Their website features educational resources, webinars, and support services for patients and their families. Website: www.liverfoundation.org

<u>Hepatitis B Information and Support Group (HBIG):</u> HBIG is an online community and support group for individuals affected by hepatitis B. It provides a platform for sharing experiences, asking questions, and connecting with others facing similar challenges. Website: www.hepbcommunity.org

<u>Hep B United:</u> Hep B United is a national coalition in the United States that aims to promote hepatitis B awareness, screening, vaccination, and linkage to care. Their website offers educational materials, advocacy resources, and information on local organizations. Website: www.hepbunited.org

<u>Hepatitis Education Project (HEP):</u> HEP is a non-profit organization based in the United States that focuses on hepatitis B and C education, support, and advocacy. Their website provides resources, fact sheets, and information on local events and support groups. Website: www.hepeducation.org

<u>British Liver Trust:</u> The British Liver Trust offers information and support for individuals with liver conditions, including hepatitis B. Their website features resources, guides, and a helpline for individuals seeking guidance and support. Website: www.britishlivertrust.org.uk

<u>Canadian Liver Foundation (CLF):</u> The CLF provides information and support for individuals with liver diseases, including hepatitis B. Their website features educational resources, publications, and a helpline for assistance and guidance. Website: www.liver.ca

It is important to note that while these resources provide reliable information and support, it is always recommended to consult with healthcare professionals for personalized advice and guidance regarding hepatitis B diagnosis, treatment, and management.

www.ingramcontent.com/pod-product-compliance
Lightning Source LLC
Chambersburg PA
CBHW072339270726
48659CB00022B/1970